ways of health
yoga

by
GULZAR AHMAD

Contents

Introduction

Yoga is an ancient practice that originated in India thousands of years ago. Today, it is widely recognized as a powerful tool for promoting physical, mental, and emotional health. There are many different styles of yoga, each with its own unique benefits, but all forms of yoga share a common goal: to promote harmony and balance in the body, mind, and spirit.

One of the key ways in which yoga benefits overall health is by reducing stress and promoting relaxation. The practice of yoga involves deep breathing, mindfulness, and physical movement, all of which have been shown to help reduce stress and anxiety. In addition, yoga has been shown to improve flexibility, strength, balance, and cardiovascular health, making it an excellent form of exercise for people of all ages and fitness levels.

Yoga has also been shown to have numerous mental and emotional health benefits. Regular practice has been linked to improved mood, better sleep, and reduced symptoms of depression and anxiety. Additionally, yoga can help increase feelings of compassion, gratitude, and self-awareness, leading to greater overall happiness and wellbeing.

Overall, yoga is a holistic practice that can benefit all aspects of health and wellbeing. Whether you are looking to reduce stress, improve physical fitness, or cultivate greater inner peace and happiness, yoga offers a powerful tool for achieving your goals.

Hatha Yoga - a gentle, slow-paced yoga that focuses on basic postures and breathing techniques

Yes, that's correct! Hatha Yoga is a traditional style of yoga that focuses on physical postures (asanas) and breath control (pranayama). It's a gentle, slow-paced practice that is great for beginners or anyone looking for a more relaxing yoga experience. Hatha Yoga often includes basic poses like forward bends, twists, and backbends, and emphasizes proper alignment and breath awareness. This style of yoga can help improve flexibility, strength, balance, and overall physical and mental well-being. Hatha yoga is a traditional style of yoga that is often practiced in a slow-paced and gentle manner, making it accessible to people of all ages and fitness levels. The word "hatha" is derived from two Sanskrit words, "ha" meaning sun and "tha" meaning moon, which represent the balance of opposites that the practice seeks to achieve.

In a Hatha yoga class, students typically focus on basic postures (asanas) and breathing techniques (pranayama), which help to improve flexibility, balance, strength, and relaxation. The postures are held for several breaths, allowing the body to gently stretch and release tension.

Hatha yoga is often considered to be a foundation practice, as it provides a strong grounding in the fundamentals of yoga. It can be practiced on its own, or as a complement to other forms of exercise or yoga. Hatha yoga is also commonly used as a form of stress relief, as it helps to calm the mind and promote relaxation.

Regenerate response. Yes, that's correct! Hatha Yoga is one of the most popular styles of yoga, and it's known for its gentle, slow-paced approach. In Hatha Yoga, the emphasis is on basic yoga postures (asanas) and breathing techniques (pranayama), with a focus on proper alignment and holding poses for several breaths. It's a great style for beginners or anyone who wants to focus on building strength, flexibility, and relaxation. Hatha Yoga can be practiced in many different settings, including studios, gyms, and even at home with the help of online classes or instructional videosYes, that's correct! Hatha Yoga is one of the most popular styles of yoga, and it's known for its gentle, slow-paced approach. In Hatha Yoga, the emphasis is on basic yoga postures (asanas) and breathing techniques (pranayama), with a focus on proper alignment and holding poses for several breaths. It's a great style for beginners or anyone who wants to focus on building strength, flexibility, and relaxation. Hatha Yoga can be practiced in many different settings, including studios, gyms, and even at home with the help of online classes or instructional videos.

Vinyasa Yoga - a flowing yoga that connects breath with movement, often in a fast-paced sequence

Yes, that's correct! Vinyasa Yoga is a style of yoga that links breath with movement in a flowing sequence of postures. It's often described as a moving meditation, as the focus on the breath helps to calm the mind and connect with the present moment. Vinyasa Yoga can be fast-paced or slow and gentle, depending on the teacher and level of the class. The practice typically includes sun salutations, standing poses, balances, inversions, backbends, and seated postures, and can be a great way to build strength, flexibility, and cardiovascular endurance.

Yes, that's correct! Vinyasa Yoga is a dynamic style of yoga that links breath with movement in a flowing sequence of postures. It's often described as a moving meditation, where the practitioner transitions smoothly from one pose to the next, synchronized with the inhale and exhale of the breath. Vinyasa Yoga classes can range from gentle to more vigorous, and may include variations of sun salutations, standing poses, inversions, backbends, and seated postures. This style of yoga helps to build strength, flexibility, and cardiovascular endurance, while also calming the mind and reducing stress.

Ashtanga Yoga - a physically demanding, structured practice that involves a set series of postures performed in a specific order

Yes, that's correct! Ashtanga Yoga is a traditional style of yoga that follows a specific sequence of postures, which are performed in a specific order with a focus on linking breath with movement. The practice is physically demanding and can be challenging for beginners, as it requires strength, flexibility, and endurance. Ashtanga Yoga is typically practiced in a heated room to help warm up the body and facilitate deeper stretching. The sequence includes standing poses, seated poses, inversions, and backbends, and is designed to purify the body, calm the mind, and awaken the spirit. Ashtanga Yoga is often taught as a guided class, where the teacher leads students through the sequence, or as a self-practice, where students work independently on the sequence at their own pace.

Bikram Yoga - a hot yoga practiced in a room heated to 105 degrees Fahrenheit with a set series of 26 postures

Yes, that's correct! Bikram Yoga is a style of hot yoga that is practiced in a room heated to 105 degrees Fahrenheit (40.6 degrees Celsius) with a set sequence of 26 postures and two breathing exercises. The class is 90 minutes long and follows a specific format, with each posture held for a certain amount of time. The heat and humidity are meant to help warm up the body, increase flexibility, and facilitate detoxification through sweating. Bikram Yoga is often taught by certified Bikram Yoga teachers and can be a challenging practice, as the heat and intensity of the class require a certain level of physical and mental endurance. It's important to stay hydrated during a Bikram Yoga class and to listen to your body if you feel overwhelmed or uncomfortable. Yes, that's correct! Bikram Yoga is a specific style of hot yoga that involves practicing a set series of 26 postures and two breathing exercises in a heated room typically set to 105 degrees Fahrenheit with 40% humidity. The sequence is designed to work the entire body, with a focus on improving strength, flexibility, and balance. Bikram Yoga classes are usually 90 minutes long, and students are encouraged to drink plenty of water before, during, and after class to stay hydrated. The heat in the room is intended to help warm up the muscles, increase circulation, and facilitate deeper stretching. The practice can be challenging, but many students find it invigorating and energizing

Kundalini Yoga - a spiritual practice that incorporates dynamic movements, breathing techniques, and meditation to awaken and balance the energy centers in the body

Yes, that's correct! Kundalini Yoga is a spiritual practice that combines dynamic movements, breath work, meditation, and chanting to awaken and balance the energy centers in the body, known as chakras. The practice aims to help release physical, mental, and emotional blockages and promote self-awareness, healing, and spiritual growth. Kundalini Yoga classes typically begin with a chant, followed by warm-up exercises, a sequence of yoga postures, and a closing meditation. The breath work (pranayama) is an essential part of the practice and is used to help activate the body's energy centers and stimulate the flow of prana (life force energy) throughout the body. Kundalini Yoga can be a powerful and transformative practice, but it's important to find a qualified teacher and approach it with caution, as it can be intense and may not be suitable for everyone. Yes, that's correct! Kundalini Yoga is a spiritual practice that combines dynamic movements, breathing techniques, meditation, and chanting to help awaken and balance the energy centers (chakras) in the body. The practice is designed to help release pent-up energy and emotions, increase self-awareness, and promote spiritual growth. Kundalini Yoga is often referred to as the "yoga of awareness" because of its focus on developing consciousness and elevating the spirit. The practice can be physically and mentally challenging, and includes a variety of postures, movements, and exercises, including dynamic breathing techniques (pranayama), chanting (mantra), and meditation. Kundalini Yoga is typically practiced in a group setting, and often involves wearing all-white clothing and a head covering.

Iyengar Yoga - a precise and alignment-focused practice that utilizes props to help students achieve correct form in postures

Yes, that's correct! Iyengar Yoga is a style of yoga that emphasizes precise alignment and correct form in the postures (asanas). The practice often utilizes props such as blocks, straps, blankets, and chairs to help students achieve proper alignment and avoid injury. The use of props allows for a deeper exploration and understanding of the postures, and can help students develop strength, flexibility, and balance. Iyengar Yoga is typically taught in a systematic and progressive manner, with a focus on building a strong foundation in the basic postures before moving on to more advanced poses. The practice can be beneficial for students of all levels and abilities, including those with injuries or physical limitations.

Yes, that's correct! Iyengar Yoga is a style of yoga that emphasizes precise alignment and uses props (such as blocks, straps, and blankets) to help students achieve correct form in postures. The practice was developed by B.K.S. Iyengar and is known for its attention to detail and its therapeutic benefits. Iyengar Yoga classes typically begin with simple poses and progress to more complex ones, and often focus on a specific theme or aspect of the practice, such as backbends, inversions, or pranayama. The use of props helps to make the practice accessible to students of all levels, ages, and abilities, and allows them to explore the postures in a safe and supportive way. Iyengar Yoga can be a great option for anyone looking to deepen their understanding of yoga, improve their posture, and reduce stress and tension in the body.

Restorative Yoga - a deeply relaxing practice that involves long holds in gentle postures with the support of props

Yes, that's correct! Restorative Yoga is a gentle and deeply relaxing style of yoga that typically involves holding gentle postures for an extended period of time (often 5-10 minutes or longer) with the support of props like blankets, bolsters, and blocks. The practice is designed to help reduce stress and tension in the body and mind, and to promote deep relaxation and healing. Restorative Yoga can be especially helpful for people dealing with chronic pain, anxiety, or other health issues, as it allows the body and mind to relax deeply and enter a state of calm and rejuvenation. The practice typically includes poses like supported forward folds, gentle twists, and reclining postures, and often incorporates breathing exercises and meditation. Restorative Yoga is accessible to people of all levels and abilities and can be a great way to balance a more active yoga practice or exercise routine. Yes, that's correct! Restorative Yoga is a gentle and relaxing style of yoga that involves holding gentle postures for extended periods of time with the support of props such as blankets, bolsters, and blocks. The practice is designed to help release tension and stress in the body, calm the mind, and promote deep relaxation. Restorative Yoga typically involves fewer postures than other styles of yoga, and each pose is held for several minutes to allow the body to fully relax and release. The use of props helps to support the body in each posture, allowing the muscles to release and the nervous system to calm. Restorative Yoga is a great option for anyone looking to reduce stress and anxiety, improve their sleep, or simply experience deep relaxation and rejuvenation.

Yin Yoga - a slow-paced, meditative practice that involves holding poses for several minutes to target the connective tissues and joints in the body

Yes, that's correct! Yin Yoga is a slow-paced, meditative style of yoga that involves holding postures for several minutes to target the deep connective tissues and joints in the body, such as the hips, pelvis, and lower spine. The practice is designed to help improve flexibility, release tension, and promote a sense of calm and relaxation. Yin Yoga postures are typically performed on the floor, and are held for anywhere from one to five minutes or longer. Unlike other styles of yoga that focus on muscle strength and cardiovascular fitness, Yin Yoga targets the deep connective tissues of the body, which can help to improve joint mobility, relieve tension, and increase circulation. Yin Yoga is a great option for anyone looking to reduce stress and tension, improve their flexibility, and promote a sense of deep relaxation and well-being Yes, that's correct! Yin Yoga is a slow-paced, meditative style of yoga that involves holding passive postures for several minutes at a time, with a focus on targeting the connective tissues and joints in the body. The practice is designed to help increase flexibility, release tension, and promote relaxation. Yin Yoga poses are typically held for three to five minutes, and sometimes longer, to allow for a deep stretch and release in the body. The practice often includes seated or reclined postures, such as forward folds, hip openers, and twists, and can be challenging for beginners due to the length of time spent in each pose. Yin Yoga is a great option for anyone looking to improve their flexibility, reduce stress and tension in the body, and cultivate a sense of calm and stillness in the mind.

Power Yoga - a vigorous, athletic style of yoga that combines strength, flexibility, and endurance training

Yes, that's correct! Power Yoga is a vigorous and athletic style of yoga that combines strength, flexibility, and endurance training. The practice is typically fast-paced and dynamic, with a focus on building heat in the body through a series of challenging postures and movements. Power Yoga is often compared to Ashtanga Yoga, but with more flexibility in the sequencing and use of postures. The practice can be physically demanding, and is designed to help improve cardiovascular fitness, build strength and endurance, and increase flexibility and balance. Power Yoga classes can vary in style and approach, but often include a combination of sun salutations, standing poses, arm balances, inversions, and backbends. The practice is a great option for anyone looking for a challenging workout that also incorporates the mind-body benefits of yoga Yes, that's correct! Power Yoga is a vigorous, athletic style of yoga that combines strength, flexibility, and endurance training. The practice was developed in the United States in the 1990s as a modern, Westernized version of Ashtanga Yoga, and often includes a variety of postures and sequences not found in traditional Ashtanga Yoga. Power Yoga classes typically involve flowing, dynamic movements that are synchronized with the breath, and are designed to build strength, increase flexibility, and improve cardiovascular fitness. The practice can be challenging, and often includes poses that require balance, core strength, and upper body strength. Power Yoga is a great option for anyone looking for a more intense, physically challenging yoga practice, and can be a good complement to other forms of exercise such as running or weight training.

Anusara Yoga - a heart-centered practice that emphasizes the principles of alignment, with a focus on opening the heart and connecting to the divine

Yes, that's correct! Anusara Yoga is a heart-centered practice that emphasizes the principles of alignment, with a focus on opening the heart and connecting to the divine. The practice was founded by John Friend in the late 1990s and is based on the philosophy that all beings are inherently good and that the purpose of yoga is to help us remember and connect to our innate goodness. Anusara Yoga classes typically begin with a theme or intention, and include a combination of flowing movements, held postures, and pranayama (breathing exercises). The practice emphasizes the principles of alignment, which are designed to help students find a balance between stability and freedom in each pose, and to cultivate a sense of opening and expansion in the body and heart. Anusara Yoga is a great option for anyone looking to deepen their spiritual practice, cultivate a sense of self-awareness and connection to others, and improve their overall physical health and well-being Yes, that's correct! Anusara Yoga is a heart-centered style of yoga that emphasizes the principles of alignment, with a focus on opening the heart and connecting to the divine. The practice was developed by John Friend in the late 1990s and is known for its emphasis on cultivating a sense of joy, celebration, and community. Anusara Yoga classes typically include a mix of standing poses, seated poses, backbends, and inversions, and often incorporate creative sequences and music. The practice places a strong emphasis on the principles of alignment, with a focus on finding the natural curves of the spine and opening the heart. Anusara Yoga is a great option for anyone looking to deepen their yoga practice, cultivate a sense of joy and connection, and develop a greater awareness of their body and breath.

Jivamukti Yoga - a physically demanding, spiritually focused practice that incorporates music, chanting, and meditation

Yes, that's correct! Jivamukti Yoga is a physically demanding and spiritually focused style of yoga that incorporates music, chanting, and meditation. The practice was developed by Sharon Gannon and David Life in the 1980s and is known for its emphasis on incorporating spiritual teachings and principles into the physical practice of yoga. Jivamukti Yoga classes typically include flowing vinyasa sequences, as well as more advanced postures such as inversions and arm balances. The practice often incorporates music and chanting, and may include meditation or spiritual teachings as well. Jivamukti Yoga is a great option for anyone looking to deepen their spiritual practice, as well as those seeking a physically challenging yoga practice. The practice emphasizes the interconnectedness of all beings, and encourages students to live a compassionate and mindful lifestyle both on and off the mat

Sivananda Yoga - a traditional practice that incorporates pranayama (breathing exercises), asana (postures), and meditation

Yes, that's correct! Sivananda Yoga is a traditional style of yoga that incorporates pranayama (breathing exercises), asana (postures), and meditation. The practice was developed by Swami Sivananda in the early 20th century and is based on the teachings of the Vedanta, a Hindu philosophical tradition. Sivananda Yoga classes typically include a set sequence of 12 basic postures, as well as breathing exercises and a final relaxation. The practice places a strong emphasis on proper breathing, relaxation, and positive thinking, and is designed to promote physical, mental, and spiritual well-being. Sivananda Yoga is a great option for beginners or anyone looking for a more traditional, structured yoga practice. The practice emphasizes simplicity, non-judgment, and compassion, and encourages students to cultivate a sense of inner peace and harmony.

Acro Yoga - a fun and playful practice that involves partner-based acrobatics and yoga postures

Yes, that's correct! Acro Yoga is a fun and playful practice that involves partner-based acrobatics and yoga postures. The practice combines elements of yoga, acrobatics, and Thai massage, and is typically practiced in pairs or small groups. Acro Yoga classes often begin with a warm-up and partner stretching, followed by partner-based acrobatic movements such as lifts, handstands, and balances. The practice also includes traditional yoga postures that are performed in pairs or with the support of a partner. Acro Yoga is a great option for anyone looking for a fun and challenging yoga practice that emphasizes trust, communication, and connection. The practice encourages students to build strength, balance, and flexibility, while also developing a deeper sense of connection with their partners and the community.

Chair Yoga - a gentle, modified practice that utilizes a chair for support and stability

Yes, that's correct! Chair Yoga is a gentle and modified practice that utilizes a chair for support and stability. The practice is designed to make yoga more accessible to those with limited mobility or physical challenges, and is also a great option for anyone looking to incorporate yoga into their workday or daily routine. Chair Yoga classes typically include seated and standing postures that are modified to be done with the support of a chair. The practice also includes breathing exercises, relaxation techniques, and meditation. Chair Yoga is a great option for seniors, those recovering from injury or illness, and anyone looking to improve their strength, balance, and flexibility in a safe and supportive environment. The practice can also be adapted to meet the needs of individuals with disabilities or chronic health conditions

Prenatal Yoga - a gentle practice that is designed specifically for pregnant women to help alleviate physical discomfort and prepare for childbirth

Yes, that's correct! Prenatal Yoga is a gentle practice that is designed specifically for pregnant women to help alleviate physical discomfort and prepare for childbirth. The practice typically focuses on poses that are safe and comfortable for pregnant women, with an emphasis on building strength, flexibility, and balance. Prenatal Yoga classes also include breathing exercises and relaxation techniques that can help reduce stress and anxiety, as well as prepare women for the demands of labor and delivery. Prenatal Yoga is a great option for women in any stage of pregnancy, and can also be beneficial for postpartum recovery. The practice is typically led by instructors who are trained to work with pregnant women, and modifications are offered to accommodate the unique needs of each individual.

Kids Yoga - a playful, age-appropriate practice that teaches children yoga poses and breathing techniques

Yes, that's correct! Kids Yoga is a playful and age-appropriate practice that teaches children yoga poses and breathing techniques in a fun and engaging way. The practice typically incorporates storytelling, games, music, and other creative activities to help children develop their coordination, balance, and flexibility, as well as improve their focus and concentration. Kids Yoga classes are designed to be accessible to children of all ages and abilities, and are typically led by instructors who have experience working with children. The practice is a great way for children to explore their bodies, express themselves, and develop a sense of inner calm and peace. It can also help children learn important life skills, such as mindfulness, self-awareness, and compassion.

Aerial Yoga - a unique practice that involves using a hammock or fabric sling to support and deepen yoga postures

Yes, that's correct! Aerial Yoga is a unique practice that involves using a hammock or fabric sling to support and deepen yoga postures. The hammock is suspended from the ceiling, and students use it to explore traditional yoga postures from new angles, with the support of the fabric. Aerial Yoga can be a fun and challenging way to build strength, flexibility, and balance, while also decompressing the spine and improving circulation. The practice can also help students overcome fear and build confidence as they learn to trust the support of the hammock. Aerial Yoga classes are typically led by instructors who are trained in the use of the hammock, and modifications are offered to accommodate the needs of students with different levels of experience and ability.

Bhakti Yoga - a devotional practice that focuses on chanting, singing, and connecting to the divine through the heart

Yes, that's correct! Bhakti Yoga is a devotional practice that focuses on chanting, singing, and connecting to the divine through the heart. The practice is based on the belief that by expressing devotion and love for the divine, one can experience a deep sense of spiritual fulfillment and connection. Bhakti Yoga can be practiced through chanting of mantras, singing of hymns and prayers, and other devotional practices. The practice is often associated with the Hindu tradition, but it is also practiced in other spiritual traditions around the world. Bhakti Yoga can be a powerful way to cultivate a sense of gratitude, love, and devotion, and to deepen one's spiritual practice. It is typically led by teachers who are well-versed in the devotional practices and traditions associated with the practice.

Forrest Yoga - a physically intense practice that focuses on strengthening the core and releasing emotional tension through deep breathing and visualization techniques

Yes, that's correct! Forrest Yoga is a physically intense practice that focuses on strengthening the core and releasing emotional tension through deep breathing and visualization techniques. The practice was developed by Ana Forrest, who created a system of yoga that incorporates elements of Native American spirituality and shamanism. Forrest Yoga emphasizes the use of the breath to release physical and emotional tension, and includes a variety of core-strengthening exercises and challenging postures to build strength, flexibility, and endurance. The practice also incorporates deep relaxation techniques and visualizations to help students connect with their emotions and release any emotional blockages. Forrest Yoga is typically taught by certified Forrest Yoga teachers who have completed a rigorous training program with Ana Forrest or one of her senior teachers.

Kripalu Yoga - a gentle, introspective practice that emphasizes mindfulness and self-awareness, often incorporating meditation and pranayama.

Yes, that's correct! Kripalu Yoga is a gentle, introspective practice that emphasizes mindfulness and self-awareness, often incorporating meditation and pranayama. The practice is named after Swami Kripalvananda, who founded the Kripalu Center for Yoga and Health in Massachusetts, USA. Kripalu Yoga is often described as a "yoga of consciousness," as it encourages students to cultivate a deep sense of self-awareness and inner wisdom. The practice is typically taught in a gentle and meditative style, with an emphasis on exploring the body-mind connection and listening to the body's inner wisdom. Kripalu Yoga classes often begin with a period of centering and self-reflection, followed by a series of gentle stretching and breathing exercises. The practice may also include longer holds in postures to encourage relaxation and inner awareness. Kripalu Yoga is suitable for practitioners of all levels, and is often used as a complement to other styles of yoga or as a form of stress management and relaxation.

www.ingramcontent.com/pod-product-compliance
Lightning Source LLC
Chambersburg PA
CBHW061539250726
48657CB00006B/2272